Nursing & Health Survival Guide

Postnatal & Neonatal Midwifery Skills

Alison Edwards

D042006B

Pearson Education Limited
Edinburgh Gate
Harlow
Essex CM20 2JE
England

and Associated Companies throughout the world

Visit us on the World Wide Web at:
www.pearson.com/uk

First published 2013

ISBN 978-0-273-76334-5

British Library Cataloguing-in-Publication Data
A catalogue record for this book is available from the British Library

Library of Congress Cataloging-in-Publication Data
A catalog record for this book is available from the Library of Congress

10 9 8 7 6 5 4 3 2 1
16 15 14 13 12

Typeset in 8/9.5pt Helvetica by 35
Printed and bound in China
EPC/01

contents

ANATOMY	1
Fetal circulation	1
Involution	3
Breast	4
BEREAVEMENT – DEALING WITH THE LOSS OF A BABY	4
BOTTLE FEEDING	6
Sterilisation of feeding equipment	6
Making up formula feeds	8
BREASTFEEDING	9
Physiology of lactation	9
Advantages of breastfeeding	11
Ten steps to successful breastfeeding	11
CALCULATING FEED REQUIREMENTS	12
CHANGING STOOLS	13
CONTRACEPTION	13
CORD CARE	18
DEVELOPMENTAL CARE	18
DISCHARGE – points for discussion	19
DRUGS FOR NEONATES	19
Vitamin K – (Phytomenadione)	19
Naloxone	20
Hepatitis B Immunoglobulin	20
BCG	20
EMERGENCIES	21
Secondary postpartum haemorrhage (PPH)	21
Sepsis	22
FLUID BALANCE	24
HAND EXPRESSION	26
HYPOGLYCAEMIA IN THE NEWBORN	28
LOCHIA	29
MEOWS – MODIFIED OBSTETRIC EARLY WARNING SYSTEM	29
NEONATAL EXAMINATION	32
NEONATAL JAUNDICE	33
Physiological jaundice	34
Pathological jaundice	35
NEONATAL SCREENING	36
Hearing tests	36
SBR – Serum Bilirubin	36
Neonatal blood spot	37
PHOTOTHERAPY	41

POST BIRTH CARE 43
  Initial general care 43
  Post instrumental 44
  Post caesarean section 44
POSTNATAL EXAMINATION 45
POSTNATAL COMPLICATIONS 46
SKIN TO SKIN 50
SUDDEN INFANT DEATH SYNDROME (SIDS) 50
THERMOREGULATION OF THE NEWBORN 51
TRANSIENT TACHYPNOEA OF THE NEWBORN 52
GENERAL ABBREVIATIONS 52
SUPPORT GROUPS 55

Anatomy

■ FETAL CIRCULATION

Figure 1 The fetal circulation

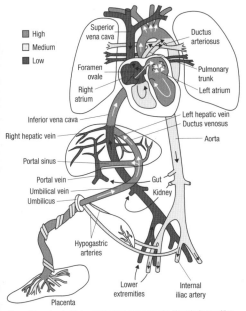

Source: Reproduced with permission from: Fernandes CJ. Physiologic transition from intrauterine to extrauterine life. In: UpToDate, Basow, DS (Ed), UpToDate, Waltham, MA 2012. Copyright © 2012 UpToDate, Inc. For more information visit www.uptodate.com

Four main structures which differ from adult circulation

- **Ductus venosus** – directs oxygenated blood from the umbilical vein to the inferior vena cava
- **Foramen ovale** – an opening between the atria of the heart which allows blood to bypass the pulmonary circulation
- **Ductus arteriosus** – diverts blood away from the pulmonary artery back into the aorta
- **Two hypogastric arteries** – direct blood from the lower extremities back through the umbilical arteries to the placenta

Extra features

- Red blood cells are greater in number and larger than adult blood cells.
- The life span of these red blood cells is shorter.
- Fetal haemoglobin has greater oxygen carrying capacity.

At birth

- Changes in temperature and compression of the chest wall during the birth stimulate the baby to take a breath.
- Blood is drawn towards the alveoli in the lungs and then returned to the left atrium of the heart. This lowers the pressure in the right atrium and raises pressure in the left atrium causing the foramen ovale to be covered by a flap of tissue. Blood is now directed into the right ventricle and out to the lungs.

- Blood bypasses the ductus arteriosus and the direction of blood circulating reverses. The ductus arteriosus eventually closes to form a ligament.
- The separation of the umbilical cord cuts off the placental blood supply further, lowering the pressure in the right atrium. Blood can no longer circulate through the hypogastric arteries, umbilical vessels and ductus venosus. These structures eventually form ligaments.

■ INVOLUTION

- The process whereby the uterus returns to its pre pregnancy size of 60 grams. By 10 days post birth the uterus is usually no longer palpable above the pelvic brim.
- **Autolysis** – proteolytic enzymes digest the muscle cells no longer required. Phagocytes remove the debris.
- **Ischaemia** – blood supply is reduced to the decidua due to constriction of the spiral arteries after birth. The decidua therefore dies and is shed as lochia. By 6 weeks post birth the endometrium has reformed.
- **Contraction and retraction** – oxytocin continues to be released (especially if the mother is breastfeeding), therefore contraction and retraction of the myometrium continues.

■ BREAST

Figure 2 The anatomy of the breast

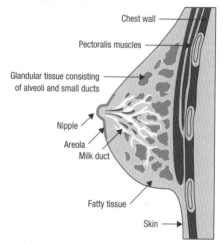

Source: http://www.celtnet.org.uk/cancer/breast-function.html

Bereavement – dealing with the loss of a baby

Unfortunately babies continue to be stillborn, die in utero or die within days of the birth. It proves to be an extremely difficult time for the families but also the staff involved. There are, however, a number of activities that need to be undertaken. Some of these may help with the emotional distress.

- Encourage though don't force the parents to hold their baby and spend some time with them – this amount of time should be dictated by the parents themselves.
- Sitting and listening/discussing events.
- Respond to the signals – every set of parents will deal differently with grief. Act professionally but sensitively and use understandable terminology.
- Take foot and hand prints, locks of hair, photographs and provide additional identity bracelets. Parents may not wish to take these away with them immediately, so store them in the notes as they may ask for them at a later date.
- Siblings need support too. Textbooks are available which provide strategies for this.
- Handle the baby gently – help the parents wash and dress their baby if they wish or do it for them.
- Discussing the funeral arrangements whilst difficult, can help provide a focus. Hospitals usually have their own policies on this and will often hold memorial services too.
- Invite faith leaders/chaplains to visit if appropriate.
- Parents often ask the question WHY it happened. It isn't always possible to answer this question but a post-mortem and a series of screening tests are offered/carried out with consent which may answer the question. An appointment to return to discuss the results with an obstetrician is required.
- All stillbirths and neonatal deaths must be reported – relevant forms will be found on each delivery suite.
- A death certificate should be completed and passed to the parents. The parents will need to register the birth and death with the Registrar of Births and Deaths within 42 days of the baby's delivery. In Scotland, the time limit

is 21 days and in Northern Ireland, the time limit is 5 days. If the parents are married, the registrar will need details of both parents. If the parents are not married, only the details of the mother are required, but the father can give his details.

- Postnatal care should continue as normal for the woman.
- Women can be offered medication to suppress lactation.
- The baby can be placed in the hospital mortuary until tests are completed and baby is collected for funeral or cremation. Until then, parents should be able to visit the baby in the chapel of rest as they wish. Alternatively, some units have refrigerated cots which enable the baby to remain with its parents.
- You will need to inform the woman's GP and cancel any referrals to the health visitors.
- Make sure that all documentation is complete.

Bottle feeding

■ STERILISATION OF FEEDING EQUIPMENT

Cold water sterilising

- Either a bought sterilising unit or a clean bucket/plastic container with a lid can be used. The bucket or container should be deep enough to submerge the equipment entirely.
- Dissolve a sterilising tablet in cold water to the suggested ratio on the packet.
- Bottles should be rinsed clear of old milk before re-sterilisation – use a bottle brush if needed.
- Submerge the bottles and teats, etc. ensuring there are no air bubbles inside.

- Use the equipment provided with the bought unit or something, such as a heavy plate, to keep the bottles and other equipment completely under the solution.
- Takes around 30 minutes to sterilise.
- Take out bottles and teats only when required. Shake out any excess solution, or rinse off the fluid with cool, boiled water (though this isn't compulsory).
- Change the solution every 24 hours.

Boiling
- Bottles should be suitable for this.
- Place in a large pan with a lid or cover. Use the pan exclusively for this purpose.
- Fill the pan with water and submerge all the feeding equipment completely. Make sure there are no trapped air bubbles inside the bottles and teats, then cover the pan and boil for at least 10 minutes.
- Keep the pan's cover on until you need to use the equipment.

Electric steam sterilising
- Takes between 8 to 12 minutes, plus cooling time.
- Can keep bottles sterilised for up to 6 hours if left in the steriliser with the lid closed.
- Bottles, teats and other equipment should be placed with their openings downwards.
- Check all equipment is safe to use in a steam steriliser before using.

Microwaves
- Check bottles can be sterilised in the microwave.
- Takes around 90 seconds to sterilise a single bottle.

- Do not seal the bottles during microwaving.
- Special steamers are available for microwave use. These steamers take about 3 to 8 minutes to work plus cooling time, depending on the model and microwave wattage.
- The items also remain sterile for 3 hours if the steriliser lid is kept closed.

Dishwasher sterilising

- Check equipment is dishwasher safe.
- Use a hot programme of 80°C or more.
- Make up feed immediately because bacteria can begin to form as soon as the bottle is removed from the dishwasher.

■ MAKING UP FORMULA FEEDS

- All equipment must have been sterilised including bottles, teats and teat covers. Leave to drip dry.
- Boil kettle and leave to cool to around 70°C (approx. 15 min for 500 ml of water).
- Wash hands thoroughly especially after changing nappies.
- ALWAYS put the correct amount of water into the bottle first.
- Using the scoop provided with the formula, add the appropriate number of scoops of milk powder. The scoops should be levelled off using a knife. The scoop must not be over or under filled.
- Place top on bottle and shake the bottle to mix the milk thoroughly.
- Allow to cool further (it should feel lukewarm to the inside of the forearm). If needed run the bottle under the cold tap.

- It is recommended that feeds should no longer be made up in advance and that any feed should be used within 2 hours. Any leftover feed should be disposed of after 2 hours.

Other tips

- Women on income support who choose to formula feed may be entitled to vouchers to get milk powder.
- Whey dominant powders are recommended over casein dominant; however, both can be used from birth.
- Babies who bottle feed are more likely to need winding post feed.
- Weaning should take place after around 6 months.

Breastfeeding

■ PHYSIOLOGY OF LACTATION

Breast changes in pregnancy

- From the sixth week of pregnancy oestrogen influences the growth of the ducts and tubules in the breast. Progesterone, prolactin and human placental lactogen (HPL) cause enlargement of the alveoli.
- By 12 weeks the Montgomery's tubercles (sebaceous glands on the areola) secrete lubricants onto the breast surface.
- Colostrum is produced under the influence of HPL and prolactin from 16 weeks gestation.
- In pregnancy milk production is inhibited by high levels of oestrogen and progesterone. These levels drop dramatically once the placenta is delivered, enabling prolactin levels to increase and milk production to commence.

Milk production

- Prolaction releasing hormone (from the hypothalamus) stimulates prolactin (from the anterior pituitary) production which in turn stimulates the acini cells of the breasts to produce milk. Prolactin release peaks towards the end of feeds.
- When suckling stops, prolactin inhibiting factor (produced by the hypothalamus and secreted in the breast milk) is released to block milk production when the feed is complete.
- Subsequently milk production works on a supply and demand principle.
- The cycle is initiated by stimulus, e.g. by the baby suckling. This stimulus results in oxytocin being released by the posterior pituitary. Oxytocin contracts the cells in the alveoli forcing milk down the milk ducts and into the baby's mouth, aided by the baby's sucking motion. (A neurohormonal reflex or the 'Let down reflex'.)

Tips

- Encouraging an initial breastfeed and skin to skin within the first hour of birth will greatly improve the success of subsequent breastfeeding.
- Prolactin levels increase at night to prepare the body for feeds the following day, so it is normal for babies to feed through the night.
- Women opting to formula feed will produce milk initially but need to avoid stimulating the breasts to aid cessation of milk production.
- Women with HIV should be discouraged from breastfeeding due to possible transmission.

■ ADVANTAGES OF BREASTFEEDING

For baby

- Protects from leukaemia, rotavirus and gastrointestinal infections
- Protects against respiratory problems including asthma and against urinary problems
- Reduces chance of developing eczema and food allergies
- Aids mouth and jaw development and teeth alignment
- Reduces the likelihood of obesity in childhood
- Reduces the risk of ear infections
- Helps prevent necrotising enterocolitis, especially in premature infants
- Thought to reduce the risk of SIDS
- Maternal antibodies are passed on to baby to aid immunity

For the woman

- Protects against breast and ovarian cancers
- May help with postmenopausal bone density
- Exclusively breastfeeding can provide effective contraception
- Aids weight loss
- Helps bonding and overall feeling of wellbeing
- Breast milk is produced on demand and at the correct temperature
- Breastfeeding is convenient and free

■ TEN STEPS TO SUCCESSFUL BREASTFEEDING

1. Units should have a written breastfeeding policy that is routinely communicated to all healthcare staff.

2. Train all healthcare staff in the skills necessary to implement the breastfeeding policy.
3. Inform all pregnant women about the benefits and management of breastfeeding.
4. Help mothers initiate breastfeeding soon after birth.
5. Show mothers how to breastfeed and how to maintain lactation even if they are separated from their babies.
6. Give newborn infants no food or drink other than breast milk, unless medically indicated.
7. Practice rooming in, allowing mothers and infants to remain together 24 hours per day.
8. Encourage breastfeeding on demand.
9. Give no artificial teats or dummies to breastfeeding infants.
10. Foster the establishment of breastfeeding support groups and refer women to them on discharge from the hospital or clinic.

Reference / WHO/UNICEF (1989) Protecting, Promoting and Supporting Breastfeeding: The special role of maternity services. A joint WHO/UNICEF Statement. Geneva: WHO.

Calculating feed requirements

Babies' feed requirements change on a daily basis.
In some cases, for example when a baby is admitted to the neonatal unit, it is necessary to calculate the correct amount for the age of the neonate. To do this the following formula is used.

$$\frac{\text{Daily requirement} \times \text{weight in kilograms}}{\text{Number of feeds in 24 hrs}}$$

Examples could be

Day 0–1 = 60 ml per day × 2 kg ÷ 8 (this will equate to 3 hourly feeds) = 10 ml per feed

Day 2 = 90 ml per day × 2 kg ÷ 6 (this equates to 4 hourly feeds) = 30 ml per feed

Day 3 = 120 ml per day × 2 kg ÷ 6 = 40 ml per feed

Changing stools

- From birth to 2 days: stool (meconium) is dark green/ black, thick and sticky.
- 3–4 days old: 'changing stools' become a less dark green/brown colour and may have 'seeds' of yellow in it.
- 5–6 days old: stool is usually yellow.
- Breastfed babies will continue to pass soft yellow, low odour stools quite frequently until about 3–4 weeks. This reduces to a bowel movement every 2–3 days after that.
- Formula fed babies are more likely to pass paler more formed stool with a slight odour. These babies are prone to constipation.

Contraception

Whilst having another baby may be the last thing on parents' minds just after giving birth, it is an important role of the midwife to discuss contraception prior to discharge.

It is entirely up to the individual couples when they resume intercourse and this can be influenced by a number of factors.

The type of contraceptive used is largely personal choice; however factors including overall health, age and lifestyle can impact on the options available.

Options available

Condoms (male)	Free from family planning centres Protects against pregnancy and Sexually Transmitted Diseases (STDs) Most have a spermicidal agent applied N.B. the majority are made of latex Can be damaged during application by nails, rings, etc. raising the risk of semen leaks
Natural methods	Can involve monitoring temperature/mucus discharge and avoidance of intercourse during fertile times Can be difficult to determine 'safe times'
Diaphragm/ cap	Must be measured and fitted Women must wait and use alternative methods until 6–8 weeks postnatal before assessment to ensure an accurate fit Should be inserted prior to intercourse and removed after 6 hours post intercourse Must be used with a spermicide to be effective

Condoms (female)	Needs to be inserted before penetration and held in place during penetration
	If used effectively can be 94% successful in preventing pregnancy and protects against STDs
Intrauterine contraceptive devices (IUCDs)	Come in a variety of shapes and sizes
	Some contain progesterone
	The copper content is toxic to sperm and ova
	Can be uncomfortable to insert especially in nulliparas women
	Post birth the woman must wait between 6–8 weeks before fitting
	Can cause an increase in bleeding initially and discomfort
	Progesterone based IUCDs also protect from uterine infection unlike other versions; however thrush is more common
	Can remain in situ for a number of years
	Strings may cause discomfort to the male during intercourse
	High success rate and easily removed

Combined pill	Tablets or patches containing oestrogen and progesterone which prevents ovulation and alters the cervical mucus Must be prescribed – taken for 21 days from start of period followed by a 7 day break for the withdrawal bleed Side effects include weight gain, headaches, mood changes and an increased risk of DVT/stroke in obese women Not recommended if breastfeeding Can be started after 21 days post birth Can be less effective if on antibiotics or have diarrhoea and vomiting, but otherwise if taken correctly is 99% effective
Progesterone only pill	Suitable for breastfeeding women Started after 21 days post birth Initially may affect the amount and frequency of periods Alters the cervical mucus inhibiting sperm transmission MUST be taken every day at around the same time therefore not suitable for women who may forget to take it. Some versions have a wider margin for missed tablets

Injected, e.g. Depo-Provera	Administered every 3 months and can lead to amenorrhoea Administered after 6 weeks postpartum if not awaiting sterilisation or have had unprotected intercourse Does not affect lactation Can lead to weight gain and depression
Implants	A rod containing slow release progesterone inserted under the skin in the upper arm under local anaesthetic Can be inserted after 21 days post birth Lasts around 3 years and has a high success rate May lead to amenorrhoea Inhibits ovulation and thickens the cervical mucus
Sterilisation	Tubal ligation (female) or vasectomy (male) Individuals require counselling as this method is permanent. Attempts to reverse these procedures are often unsuccessful. Usually undertaken at least 6–8 weeks following birth Small failure rate
Exclusive breastfeeding	The baby must be totally breastfed Effective in the first 6 months post birth The woman should be amenorrhoeic

Cord care

- The umbilical stump will harden and dry through a process of dry gangrene. This is helped by exposure to air.
- As the cord separates (within about 10 days), there may be some sticky residue at the base, which is normal.
- Current evidence recommends leaving the cord outside of the nappy (fold the top of the nappy down) and leave alone.
- At most, use clean water and cotton wool to remove any contamination.
- Do not apply any powders or creams.
- The cord clamp may or may not be removed once the cord has dried – this depends on Trust policy.

Developmental care

- Complements the high-tech medical and nursing care that occurs on neonatal units.
- Provides care around the needs of the individual.
- Based on the principle of recreating features of the intrauterine environment including – controlled light and sound, diurnal rhythms, constant temperature, nutrition, tactile and vestibular input (uterine boundaries support posture, tone and movement, calming behaviour).
- Light and noise exposure are kept to a minimum.
- Regular contact with parents is important – massage, touching, holding, kangaroo care are encouraged.
- Adequate pain relief is important.
- Careful positioning in a secure environment.
- Environmental temperature is regulated.

Discharge – points for discussion

It is recommended that certain topics are discussed with women prior to their leaving the hospital following their birth. Different trust policies may vary but these topics could include:

- Baby car safety
- Registering the birth – usually required within 42 days of the birth
- Contraception
- Emergency contact numbers
- Infant feeding
- Follow up visits including a six week appointment (usually with the GP)
- Signs of deviations from normal

Drugs for neonates

■ VITAMIN K – (PHYTOMENADIONE)

- Given either through midwives exemption (NMC 2011) or prescribed by a paediatrician. Premature babies or babies below 2.5 kg must have a prescription due to a greater risk of kernicterus (British National Formula 2009).
- At birth babies are deficient in vitamin K and are at risk of haemorrhage including intracranial bleeding, hence administration.
- Consent must be obtained from the parents.
- IM dose – single dose 1 mg (0.1 ml) after birth

or

- Oral × 1 dose of 2 mg (0.2 ml) at birth and at 7 days. A third dose is recommended for breastfed babies at 28 days.

- With oral administration there is a risk that babies will spit out some of the medicine, or some may not be absorbed, potentially making it less effective.
- The IM route can cause pain and swelling at the administration site.
- Little evidence is available to support a link between childhood leukaemia and the IM administration of vitamin K.

■ NALOXONE

- No longer in regular use.
- Reversal of neonatal respiratory depression arising from opioid administration to a woman in labour.
- IM injection of 200 micrograms or 10 micrograms/kg. Second doses may be needed due to a short half-life.
- Contraindicated in women who use opioids for recreational purposes.
- Can be given via midwives exemptions or prescribed.

■ HEPATITIS B IMMUNOGLOBULIN

- Administered IM. 200 units as soon after birth as possible to babies of mothers with Hepatitis B during pregnancy or are positive for Hepatitis B surface antigen.
- Is considered within the midwives exemptions (NMC 2011); however, review trust policy.

■ BCG

- Administered to babies at risk of exposure, e.g. with parents from a high risk country.
- Intradermal injection of 0.1 ml.
- Training is required to administer and needs prescribing by a medical practitioner.

Emergencies

■ SECONDARY POSTPARTUM HAEMORRHAGE (PPH)

- Occurs after 24 hours of birth and up to 6 weeks postpartum.
- Relatively uncommon.

Figure 3 Management of a secondary postpartum haemorrhage

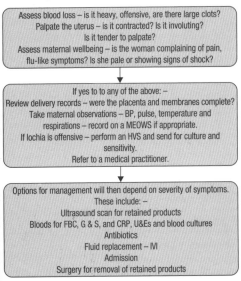

Assess blood loss – is it heavy, offensive, are there large clots?
Palpate the uterus – is it contracted? Is it involuting?
Is it tender to palpate?
Assess maternal wellbeing – is the woman complaining of pain, flu-like symptoms? Is she pale or showing signs of shock?

↓

If yes to to any of the above: –
Review delivery records – were the placenta and membranes complete?
Take maternal observations – BP, pulse, temperature and respirations – record on a MEOWS if appropriate.
If lochia is offensive – perform an HVS and send for culture and sensitivity.
Refer to a medical practitioner.

↓

Options for management will then depend on severity of symptoms.
These include: –
Ultrasound scan for retained products
Bloods for FBC, G & S, and CRP, U&Es and blood cultures
Antibiotics
Fluid replacement – IVI
Admission
Surgery for removal of retained products

- Concluding how much blood loss is considered to be a 2°PPH is subjective. Management will depend on maternal wellbeing, and whether blood loss is greater than average with or without clots.
- Most common causes are retained products of conception (RPOC), sub involution of the uterus or uterine infection.

■ SEPSIS

For more details refer to Centre for Maternal and Child Enquiries

- **Sepsis is now the leading cause of maternal deaths in the UK. Prompt recognition and actions in response to signs and symptoms is recommended.**
- **β Haemolytic Streptococcus A infection was the leading cause of the sepsis resulting in maternal deaths.**

Reference / CMACE (2011) *Saving Mothers' Lives: Reviewing maternal deaths to make motherhood safer: 2006–2008.*

Signs requiring urgent referral by ambulance
- Pyrexia >38°C – however, hypothermia may also be a sign
- Continued tachycardia >100 bpm
- Increased respiration rate/breathlessness
- Abdominal or chest pain
- Diarrhoea and vomiting – can be misdiagnosed as other conditions, e.g. gastroenteritis
- Uterine pain/tenderness
- The woman is feeling unwell, over anxious

- Leucopenia $<4 \times 10^9$ white blood cells is significant
- Persistent bleeding and offensive lochia

N.B. Anti-pyrexial medication can mask a high temperature therefore doesn't exclude sepsis.

Recommendations

- Educate women regarding the signs and symptoms.
- Women should wash hands before and after using the toilet, changing pads or touching any perineal wounds. This is increasingly important if the woman has been in contact with anyone with a sore throat or has one herself.
- Staff should be trained in the recognition of symptoms and the need for early management.

Management

- Refer to hospital/medical practitioner ASAP.
- If infection is suspected – USS for retained products +/– evacuation of retained products.
- FBC, CRP and blood cultures if temperature >38°C.
- Throat swabs, high vaginal swab, wound swabs.
- Any other relevant samples, e.g. MSU, sputum, breast milk, perineum, wound.
- Commence intravenous high dose, broad spectrum antibiotics without waiting for microbiology results. Change to appropriate antibiotics once pathogen identified. Continue for 7–10 days.
- Baby may also require surface swabs.
- Regularly record vital signs – commence MEOWS and fluid balance chart.
- Ensure baby is cared for or transferred with mother.

Septic shock

Arterial hypertension that is refractory to fluid resuscitation (CMACE 2011). Fluid overload can lead to fatal pulmonary or cerebral oedema and should therefore be avoided.

Senior anaesthetic input is vital alongside liaison with a critical care team.

Clear accurate records of fluid balance is vital!

Fluid balance

Fluid balance is maintaining the correct amount of fluid in the body through the amount of fluid intake and that which is excreted.

Around 52% of the body weight is from fluid in a non-pregnant woman. During pregnancy an increase in circulating volume of up to 50% alongside retention of fluid leading to oedema, can affect fluid balance. There are a number of factors that will cause fluid loss and gain in childbearing women:

Loss
- Vomiting, e.g. during labour or from hyperemesis in pregnancy
- Blood loss from the birth, perineal trauma or operative procedures
- Sweating/fever
- Haemorrhage, e.g. postpartum haemorrhage
- Diarrhoea

Gain
- Oedema/fluid retention
- Pre-eclampsia/eclampsia

- Renal failure
- High sodium intake
- Over infusion of intravenous fluids

Recording fluid balance

Recording fluid balance is usually required for women who are on a high dependency unit, for example, due to pre-eclampsia or those who have undergone a caesarean section/surgery.

It is usually undertaken alongside vital observations including blood pressure, pulse, respiration and temperature. High risk women may also have a Central venous pressure (CVP) line sited for more accurate measurements of circulatory function. (CVP is a measurement of pressure in the right atrium of the heart.) These measurements can alter in response to fluid loss or gain, e.g. too little circulating fluid will lead to a weak thready pulse.

Alongside the above – accurate recordings on a fluid balance chart of all fluids in and out is required. Output of urine is relatively easy to measure especially if a catheter is in situ. Urine may be measured 1 hourly or every time the catheter bag is emptied. Alternatively women can use a bedpan or bowl to collect any urine passed. Measuring input is less straightforward. Drinking vessels can vary considerably in size therefore finding out the correct volume is important. Cans and bottled fluids usually have the volume on the packaging. Most intravenous fluids are administered via pumps or have a specified amount prescribed.

Blood tests such as urea and electrolytes, glucose, magnesium and calcium can also indicate whether there are any fluid balance problems.

The totals for input and output should be calculated after a 12 or 24 hour period. The two resulting figures should be relatively the same. Marked discrepancies must be acted on.

Pre-eclamptic women are at particular risk of fluid retention. It may be necessary to restrict their fluid intake to 85 ml/hr. This includes any infused fluids, oral fluids and any medication administered in liquid form.

Hand expression

Figure 4 Hand expression

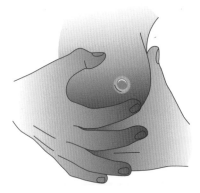

Where women are unable to directly breastfeed their babies, for example if the baby is on the neonatal unit, hand expression is recommended. If possible this should take place 6–8 times during a 24 hour period, including the night. This skill can take some practice but can prove more effective than using breast pumps and is said to produce milk with a higher fat content.

Procedure

- Wash hands (and the breasts if needed – some nipple creams need to be wiped away).
- A sterilised container wide enough to sit under the breast to collect the milk is required.
- The woman should be sitting comfortably, well supported and as upright as possible.
- To aid the release of oxytocin either have baby nearby, or ask the woman to gently massage each breast for about 5 minutes each. Using warm flannels may also help.
- Ask the woman to place her little finger underneath her breast, against her ribs, and use the remaining fingers to support the breast. The thumb needs to be on top, about 2 cm or 4 cm back from the base of the nipple, depending on breast size and shape. The woman should be feeling for a change in the texture of the breast.
- The hand should be pushed inwards towards the chest wall and the fingers should gently compress the breast tissue in a press and release motion towards the nipple.
- This rhythmic motion should be repeated until drops of colostrum or breast milk appear at the nipple. **N.B.** It may take a minute or two for milk to appear.

- DO NOT drag the fingers and thumb over the skin of the breast, as this may cause damage to the skin.
- Systematically reposition the hand slightly and repeat the movement on different sections of the breast before changing to the other breast.

Breast milk storage

- Milk should be refrigerated as soon as possible but can be kept up to 6 hours at room temperature in a sealed sterile container.
- Can be kept towards the back of a fridge for up to 5 days.
- Can be kept in a freezer for 3–6 months and in a deep freezer for up to a year.
- Any defrosted milk should not be refrozen.

Reference / For further information, see leaflet on *Expression and Storing Breast Milk*, by The Breastfeeding Network available at http://www.breastfeedingnetwork.org.uk/pdfs/BFNExpressing&Storing.pdf

Hypoglycaemia in the newborn

- More likely in babies who have IUGR or diabetic mothers, are pre term or have suffered fetal distress.
- A blood sugar of <2.6 mmol/L is considered low.
- Signs include poor tone, mottled pale skin, lethargy, poor feeding, jittering – if severe or prolonged can lead to cyanosis, hypoxia or death.

Management

- Feed immediately, and at regular intervals after that, e.g. 2–3 hourly.
- Blood sugar samples should be taken 1 hour after each feed.
- Refer to a paediatrician.
- Document.

Lochia

- The vaginal loss following the birth.
- 3–4 days post birth = RUBRA (red from blood from placental site, decidual tissue, vernix and amniotic fluid).
- 5–9 days post birth = SEROSA (pink then brown from reduced blood loss, serum and leucocytes).
- 10–28 days post birth = ALBA (yellow/white from cervical mucus, debris and leucocytes).

MEOWS – Modified Obstetric Early Warning System

- Designed for use on all women but especially those who are high risk.
- Designed to alert staff to act on any deviations from the normal.
- Regular observations including vital signs are plotted and any results falling outside accepted ranges (in some cases within the amber or red sections or in some cases a score) should trigger a referral to medical staff.

Figure 5 MEOWS chart

CHAPTER 19 ANNEX A

OBSTETRIC EARLY WARNING CHART. FOR MATERNITY USE ONLY

NAME: ____________________ DOB: ____________

CHI: WARD:

NHS Forth Valley

CONTACT DOCTOR FOR EARLY INTERVENTION IF PATIENT TRIGGERS ONE RED OR TWO YELLOW SCORES AT ANY ONE TIME

	Date:																		
	Time:																		
RESP (write rate in corresp. box)	>30																		>30
	21–30																		21–30
	11–20																		11–20
	0–10																		0–10
Saturations	90–100%																		90–100%
	< 90%																		<90%
02 Conc.	%																		%
Temp ■	39																		39
	38																		38
	37																		37
	36																		36
	35																		35
HEART RATE ■	170																		170
	160																		160
	150																		150
	140																		140
	130																		130
	120																		120
	110																		110
	100																		100
	90																		90
	80																		80
	70																		70
	60																		60
	50																		50
	40																		40

Systolic blood pressure	180, 170, 160, 150, 140, 130, 120, 110, 100, 90, 80, 70, 60, 50
Diastolic blood pressure	130, 120, 110, 100, 90, 80, 70, 60, 50, 40
Passed Urine	Y or N
Lochia	Normal / Heavy/Foul
Proteinuria	2+ / >2+
Liquor	Clear/Pink / Green
NEURO RESPONSE (√)	Alert / Voice / Pain/Unresponsive
Pain Score (no.)	2–3 / 0–1
Nausea (√)	YES (√) / NO (√)
Looks unwell (√)	YES (√) / NO (√)
Total Yellow Scores	
Total Red Scores	

Source: Adapted from Dr Fiona McIlveney and Dr Chris Cairns, NHS Forth Valley. Reproduced with permission

Neonatal examination

Alongside the initial examination after birth and the check undertaken by the paediatric team (or appropriately trained midwife) babies are regularly examined during the postnatal period. This usually takes place during the same visits as the postnatal check for the mother.

Procedure

- Make sure the examination takes place in a warm, draught-free environment and in good light.
- Gain consent from the mother and wash hands.
- If in hospital – check there are two identity labels and security bracelet in situ.
- Assess overall wellbeing – tone, response to handling, alertness.
- Discuss feeding patterns with the mother.
- Assess for any jaundice.
- Check the eyes for any discharge – take a swab if appropriate.
- Examine the mouth for any signs of infection, e.g. white spots may be sign of oral thrush.
- Check the skin for any rashes, bruises, marks.
- Examine the cord/umbilical area. Is the cord on or off, dry not sticky? There should be no odour or inflammation. If needed take a swab. Advise the mother to keep the nappy off the cord, especially in boys, to minimise contamination from urine and faeces. Remove cord clamp as per Trust policy.
- Examine the nappy area for any soreness.

- Discuss with the mother about the frequency of wet and soiled nappies and colour of the stool passed.
- Weigh baby if appropriate – newborn babies will commonly lose up to 10% of their birth weight during the first 7 days. Any greater weight loss or continued weight loss must be followed up.
- Undertake any neonatal screening as required – in some Trusts a baby's Pulse oximetry is conducted whilst in hospital.
- Support parents with any baby care queries, e.g. changing nappies, cord care, bathing baby.
- Document findings.

Reference / Ewer, A.K., Middleton, L.J., Furmston, A.F. et al. (2011) Pulse oximetry screening for congenital heart defects in newborn infants (PulseOx): a test accuracy study. Published online 5 Aug www.thelancet.com

Neonatal jaundice – physiological and pathological

Jaundice is the most common condition that may require medical attention in newborns. Jaundice is the result of accumulation of unconjugated bilirubin which leads to yellow coloration of the skin and mucous membranes. In most infants, this is not a problem but in some infants serum bilirubin levels may rise excessively, which can be harmful. Unconjugated bilirubin is neurotoxic and can, if excessive and not treated, cause death in newborns and lifelong neurologic problems in infants who survive. These babies may develop kernicterus.

Physiology (a brief description)

Neonatal jaundice develops as a result of the breakdown of the excess fetal red blood cells, no longer required after birth, into haem and globin. There is also a simultaneous change of cell haemoglobin from fetal to adult haemoglobin. The haem component is reduced into unconjugated bilirubin, which is fat soluble and requires proteins to transport it to the liver for disposal. If this protein is absent there is a risk that unconjugated bilirubin can remain in the circulation and cross into the brain.

If proteins are present, the unconjugated bilirubin is transported to the liver and converted by enzymes into water soluble bilirubin. This is transported to the small intestine via the bile ducts, followed by the colon. The waste products from this process are excreted in the urine and faeces giving them their colour.

■ PHYSIOLOGICAL JAUNDICE

At birth the liver is immature and intestinal function is decreased until feeding is established. Subsequently breastfed babies may be more prone to longer periods of jaundice (Breastfeeding jaundice).

The degree of jaundice can also be affected by gestational age and also the degree of trauma suffered at birth. Bruising from an instrumental birth, for example, can further increase the amount of bilirubin produced.

Signs and symptoms

- Develops from around day 3.
- Slowly disappears after 5 days.

- Baby is usually well and feeding regularly.
- Generally begins on the face and spreads downwards.
- Yellow coloration of the sclera of the eyes and mucous membranes, e.g. gums.

Assessment and management

- Explore history of birth, pregnancy, etc. for any predisposing factors.
- Examination should be conducted in good natural light.
- Assess overall wellbeing – tone, alertness, bowel and bladder function.
- Examine the face, body skin, gums and tongue for yellowing (consider ethnicity).
- Obtain a capillary serum bilirubin sample if considered appropriate. If high then treatment may be required – see section on phototherapy.
- Management depends on severity – monitor and review regularly/ screen/transfer/ treat.
- Educate parents about signs and symptoms.
- If baby is otherwise well – regulate feeds to 3–4 hourly; waking baby if required.
- Supplementary feeds or extra fluids are NOT recommended for breastfed babies.

■ PATHOLOGICAL JAUNDICE

- Possible causes include – haemolytic disease, rhesus disease, ABO incompatibility, genetic links.
- Increased risk for premature babies or those with underlying conditions.
- Develops within the first 2 days of life.

- High levels of unconjugated bilirubin develop and can lead to kernicterus.
- Needs immediate referral and treatment.

Signs of Kernicterus
- Hypotonia followed by, poor sucking reflex, poor feeding
- Lethargy, unresponsiveness
- Fitting
- Irritability/high pitched cry
- Back arching
- Vomiting

Neonatal screening

■ HEARING TESTS

Hearing problems are estimated to affect 1–3:1000 babies. It is recommended that all newborn babies are now given a hearing test prior to discharge from hospital or have the test as soon as possible when home. The two non-invasive tests (the oto-acoustic emission and automated auditory brainstem response test) measure emissions of low level inaudible sounds from the inner ear. The benefit of such early screening lies in the early intervention of speech therapy in those found to have hearing impairment.

■ SBR – SERUM BILIRUBIN

A capillary blood sample, from the baby's heel, which tests for the level of serum bilirubin. The result is plotted on a graph and a decision made whether to use phototherapy or not. (Please see the jaundice and phototherapy sections.) Once taken, the sample should be labelled and covered before being forwarded to the laboratory. This minimises the exposure to light which causes the breakdown of the bilirubin content, leading to an inaccurate result.

■ NEONATAL BLOOD SPOT

- Originally known as the Guthrie test.
- Undertaken between 5–8 days when feeding is more established. (Day of birth is counted as day 0.)
- Screens for all or some of the following – phenylketonuria (PKU), congenital hypothyroidism (CHT), cystic fibrosis (CF), altered haemoglobins, e.g. sickle cell, and MCADD (medium-chain acyl-CoA dehydrogenase deficiency).
- Post to laboratory within 24 hours of sample being taken.
- For more information refer to Standards and Guidelines for Newborn Blood Spot Screening (2008) UK Newborn Screening Programme Centre. www.newbornbloodspot.screening.nhs.uk

Note The Blood Spot Card is periodically updated; go to following link for the current version in use www.newbornbloodspot.screening.nhs.uk/bloodspotcard

Figure 6 Sample Blood Spot Card

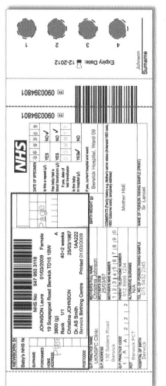

Procedure

- Obtain and document consent from the parents.
- Complete all boxes on the card and apply baby's barcode label (when available). If label is unavailable the NHS number MUST be written on the card.
- Avoid contamination when completing the card.
- Ensure that the baby is held either by a parent or the midwife, in a secure position. Having the legs hanging downwards can help blood flow. Breastfeeding during the procedure can alleviate some distress.
- Clean and warm the heel. Use a warm towel or pad, DO NOT immerse in hot water to avoid risk of scalding.
- Wash hands and put on gloves.
- Using an automated lancet, prick the heel once. A repeat stab (in a different place) should only be performed if bleeding is insufficient.
- Heel puncture should be performed on the plantar surface of the heel as shown in Figure 7 to minimise trauma.
- Wait up to 15 seconds to allow blood to flow.
- Apply the blood drop to one side of the card. Do not touch the foot onto the card.
- Allow the blood to fill the circle by natural flow, and seep through to the back. Fill the circle completely and avoid layering.
- Wipe excess blood from the heel and apply gentle pressure to the wound with cotton wool to stem bleeding. Apply a spot plaster and advise the parents to remove it no later than 24 hours afterwards or immediately if any signs of an allergic reaction occurs.
- Dispose of sharps and clinical waste.
- Remove gloves and wash hands.

Figure 7 Position for obtaining blood samples from babies

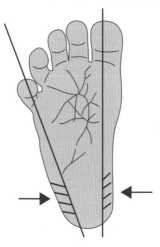

- Sign the form and insert into the envelopes provided. Post the card within 24 hours.
- Document test number and date in the postnatal records.
- Inform the parents about how they would hear about the results. Results are sent usually through to GP clinics or health visitors who will transfer the results to the 'red book'. If any abnormalities are detected the parents will be contacted via the hospital and the baby brought back for repeat tests.

> *Tip* If bleeding stops during the procedure firmly wipe
> across the puncture site with gauze or cotton wool.
> Only if needed repeat the puncture with a clean lancet
> on a different part of the foot.

Phototherapy

Bilirubin is altered by exposure to light. Therefore exposing a
jaundiced baby to light will aid the breakdown of harmful
unconjugated bilirubin.

Phototherapy will be commenced when blood serum levels
of bilirubin are high. This is determined using graphs such as
in Figure 8.

- Equipment can either produce blue or white wave light
  with different effects.
- Overhead units or specially designed cots can be used.
  Extreme jaundice may require double phototherapy or
  even require a blood exchange transfusion.
- Side effects can include raised temperature, watery stools,
  retinal damage, rashes and dehydration.

Care of a baby undergoing phototherapy

- The light source MUST be a safe distance from the baby
  (screens/head shields will be used).
- Baby's eyes should remain covered with goggles
  whenever the light source is on.
- Regular monitoring of baby's temperature.
- Baby is likely to be nursed naked except for a nappy.
- Regular checks of serum bilirubin. Turn lights off to take
  sample.

Figure 8 Phototherapy graph

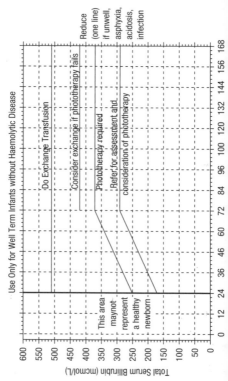

Use Only for Well Term Infants without Haemolytic Disease

- Maintain hygiene especially around nappy and cord areas in light of frequency of passing loose stools.
- Prevent infection.
- Encourage bonding with parents whenever possible – provide reassurance.

Post birth care

■ INITIAL GENERAL CARE (In no particular order)

- Provide adequate analgesia.
- Stop any infusions when permitted to do so.
- Remove any cannulas and epidural tubing when safe to do so.
- Assist with hygiene – help into the shower/bedbath.
- Assist with initial feed – encourage skin to skin even if not intending to breastfeed.
- Ensure urine is passed within 4 hours post birth.
- Assess vital signs – BP, pulse, temperature – frequency will depend on maternal wellbeing and mode of delivery.
- Palpate the uterus to ensure it is contracted.
- Provide refreshments.
- Check blood loss per vagina.
- Repair any perineal trauma and monitor regularly during the postnatal period.
- Check if bloods are required for Kliehauer if rhesus negative. Administer Anti D if required within the first 72 hours post birth.
- Educate the woman about reporting any problems.
- Answer any questions.
- Document findings.
- Act on any deviations from normal.

■ POST INSTRUMENTAL

As above plus:

- Stronger analgesia may be required due to the greater likelihood of perineal trauma and discomfort.
- Physiotherapy referral may be appropriate to discuss postnatal exercises.

■ POST CAESAREAN SECTION

As above plus:

- Ensure airway remains patent especially if post general anaesthetic.
- Continue oxygen therapy as prescribed.
- Referral to a physiotherapist to discuss breathing and abdominal exercises.
- Monitor the wound site for any oozing/bleeding. Apply a pressure dressing if needed.
- If a drain is in situ ensure it is working correctly.
- Maintain a MEOWS chart and fluid balance chart.
- Provide adequate analgesia.
- Encourage mobility as soon as possible.
- It is likely that an Intravenous infusion and catheter are in situ which need monitoring and care.
- Gradually introduce fluids, then diet according to maternal condition.
- Apply elastic support stockings if not already in situ.
- Administer any prescribed heparin and/or antibiotics.
- Assist with caring for baby as less mobile.

Postnatal examination

After the initial care post birth regular examinations are undertaken.

- Read notes and birth summary.
- Wash hands and put on apron.
- Consider mental wellbeing – talk about how the woman is feeling/coping.
- Observe the woman for general wellbeing – does she look pale, tired, unwell.
- Take vital signs – BP, pulse, respirations and temperature (the frequency of future recordings will depend on maternal condition and trust policy).
- Discuss method of feeding – discuss how breasts feel, e.g. are they engorged, tender, or has she got cracked nipples?
- Gently palpate the uterus to check it is contracted and involuting.
- Discuss the amount of vaginal loss. Ask to see the pads if concerned (see Lochia section).
- If any perineal trauma occurred, visualise the wound site. Look for signs of inflammation, stickiness, infection.
- If post Caesarean section – examine wound for signs of healing. (Remove sutures/clips if and when appropriate.)
- Discuss bladder function. If policy, collect and measure the first urine output following the birth.
- Discuss bowel function. Constipation can be common following a birth especially if taking regular analgesia.
- Examine legs for any signs of thrombosis or excessive oedema.
- Record all findings in postnatal notes/MEOWS charts.
- Act on any deviations from normal.

Postnatal complications

COMPLICATION	COMMENTS
Breast engorgement	• Occurs as milk production takes over from colostrum production. More milk than can be stored in the acini cells is initially produced, which leaks into the surrounding breast tissue
	• Occurs in all women following childbirth irrespective of feeding method, from around day 3
	• Women may experience discomfort and develop a pyrexia
	• Mild analgesia such as Paracetamol × 1 gram can help with both of these symptoms. (No more than 8 tablets in 24 hours)
	• Women should wear a well-fitting and supportive bra
	• If ceasing breastfeeding, avoidance of breast stimulation is beneficial. Otherwise encouraging the baby to feed will help
	• If heavily engorged women may find attaching baby to the breast more difficult. Hand expressing a small amount of milk should soften the breast to aid attachment
	• The use of cabbage leaves and hot/cold flannels is not supported by scientific evidence; however, women sometimes find them of benefit

Sore/cracked nipples	• Usually due to incorrect attachment during feeds • Check the baby's attachment and reposition if needed • Creams may relieve some of the discomfort between feeds
Mastitis	• Usually occurs due to inadequate emptying of the breast, alongside pressure from an incorrectly attached baby or ill-fitting bra. Blockages in the milk ducts can become infected leading to pain, redness and lumps forming • Feeding baby regularly and ensuring correct attachment will help • If the symptoms persist then antibiotics may be required
Pain/perineal discomfort	• The degree of pain depends on the individual and the mode of birth/degree of any trauma • Mild analgesics, e.g. Paracetamol, if taken regularly, can help and most are safe if breastfeeding. Stronger analgesics and anti-inflammatories can be prescribed where appropriate • In some situations cold packs can be useful. Bathing in warm water can also be soothing for perineal discomfort and will maintain hygiene • Avoidance of perfumed soaps etc. and undertaking pelvic floor exercises will promote wound healing along with a healthy diet and adequate fluid intake • Uterine pain or painful stitches accompanied by inflammation or signs of infection must be followed up • To minimise the risks of Sepsis women should be encouraged to wash their hands before and after changing pads and using the toilet

COMPLICATION	COMMENTS
Deep vein thrombosis	• Childbearing women have a much higher risk of developing a DVT • Most commonly situated in the legs • Signs and symptoms include – localised swelling, inflammation and pain • There is an increased risk of a clot travelling to the lungs, leading to pulmonary embolism – signs include – breathlessness and chest pain • Refer to a medical practitioner as soon as symptoms develop • Prevention is best – encourage leg exercises, mobility, weight loss if needed and fluid intake. Elastic support stockings can help. Avoid long journeys.
Urinary tract problems	• A degree of stress incontinence in the first few days following the birth is relatively common • Urinary tract infections should be ruled out if symptoms of frequency, burning or pain on micturition occur. (Note: urine will be mixed with lochia; therefore if obtaining a midstream sample, ask the woman to wash the vulval area thoroughly prior to collection) • Encourage fluid intake – aim for 2 litres of fluid per day • Women should be encouraged to void urine within 4 hours of the birth or removal of a catheter. The amount of urine passed should be recorded

COMPLICATION	COMMENTS
'Baby blues'	<ul><li>Many women experience these from around the third to the tenth day postpartum</li><li>Usually self-limiting</li><li>Women can complain of tiredness, tearfulness and irritability</li><li>Extra reassurance and support from the midwife and family can help</li></ul>
Postnatal depression	<ul><li>Can begin with signs of the 'baby blues'</li><li>Other symptoms include anxiety, lethargy, difficulty sleeping and feelings of guilt</li><li>Women with a history of depression, from low socioeconomic status or women who have experienced a traumatic labour and birth, are more at risk of postnatal depression</li><li>Requires referral as soon as possible</li></ul>
Puerperal psychosis	<ul><li>Least common mental health condition, affecting around 1:500 women</li><li>Sudden onset after a period of feeling well</li><li>Women can demonstrate obsessional thoughts, e.g. their baby is dead</li><li>Immediate referral is needed</li></ul>

Skin to skin

- Aim to initiate skin to skin within the first hour of birth to aid bonding and breastfeeding.
- Helps with maintaining baby's temperature and regulation of the heartbeat.
- Can be undertaken by either parent.
- Especially beneficial for premature babies (kangaroo care).
- The baby should have direct skin to skin contact and then be covered with warm towels or blankets.

Sudden Infant Death Syndrome (SIDS)

Advice to parents

- Never smoke in the same room as the baby – preferably stop smoking. This includes both parents and family members.
- Baby should sleep on its back only. To avoid flattening the occiput and problems with hip development parents are encouraged to keep the head in the midline when in a car seat and encourage play periods with baby on its stomach.
- The baby's feet should be against the bottom of the cot.
- When indoors do not cover baby's head.
- Avoid baby overheating – add or remove single layers of natural fibre clothes if feeling cold or hot. Test the temperature by feeling the back of the neck or the abdomen rather than the forehead.
- Aim to have baby sleeping in its parents room for the first six months.
- Avoid sleeping in bed or on a chair with baby, especially if under the influence of drugs, prescribed medication which could cause drowsiness or alcohol.

- If baby seems unwell seek medical help straight away.
- Breastfeed.
- Mattresses in cots should be of appropriate standard.
- Avoid using cot bumpers, duvets and pillows when baby is actually using the cot.

Thermoregulation of the newborn

Babies are at greater risk of losing heat due to a high surface area to body ratio, an immature heat regulatory centre, inability to shiver and low store of body fat. A low temperature will also impact on the baby's ability to control its blood sugar. Babies with hypoglycaemia are often hypothermic too.

Routes of heat loss
- EVAPORATION – through moisture loss from wet skin
- CONVECTION – heat drawn off by cool air passing over the skin
- CONDUCTION – via direct contact with a cold surface
- RADIATION – heat being lost to colder surfaces in close vicinity

Avoid heat loss
- Shut windows and doors, turn off fans during the birth and when performing any examinations to prevent draughts.
- Thoroughly dry baby at birth and quickly dry after bathing.
- Do not place a baby directly onto cold surfaces, e.g. weighing scales. Use warm towels.
- Best of all use skin to skin with mum or dad.

Transient tachypnoea of the newborn (TTN)

Occurs when the fluid found in the lungs in utero takes longer than expected to clear.

Symptoms
- Flaring of the nostrils
- 'Grunting'
- Sternal recession

Action
- Refer to paediatrician
- Observe and monitor for cyanosis
- Screen for infection (surface swabs) if requested
- Keep warm/monitor temperature
- A capillary blood sugar may be requested

General abbreviations

> *Tip* Many abbreviations are used in midwifery; however, officially only those accepted by your individual Trust should be used!

APH	antepartum haemorrhage
BD	twice daily
BMI	body mass index
BP	blood pressure
BPM	beats per minute
C/O	care of/complaining of
CAF	Common Assessment Framework
CRL	crown rump length

CTG	cardiotocograph
DOB	date of birth
DV	domestic violence
DVT	deep vein thrombosis
EDD	estimated due date/estimated date of delivery
EBL	estimated blood loss
FBC	fluid balance chart or full blood count
FBS	fetal blood sample
FD	forceps delivery
FH	fundal height
FHHR	fetal heart heard and regular/reactive
FL	femur length
FM	fetal movements
FSE	fetal scalp electrode
G	gravida (the number of pregnancies)
G & S	group and save
H/O	history of
Hb	haemoglobin
HC	head circumference
HELLP	haemolysis, elevated liver enzymes and low platelets
HVS	high vaginal swab
IUCD	intrauterine contraceptive device
IUD	intrauterine death
IUGR	intrauterine growth restriction
IVI	intravenous Infusion
LBW	low birth weight
LFT	liver function tests
LOA	left occipito anterior
LOP	left occipito posterior
LSCS	lower segment caesarean section

MC & S	microscopy and sensitivity
MEW/MEOW	modified early (obstetric) warning score
ML	millilitre
MLC	midwifery led care
MSU	mid stream urine
NBM	nil by mouth
NG	nasogastric
NNU	neonatal unit
NVB	normal vaginal birth
OA	occipito anterior
OP	occipito posterior
P	parity (the number of births over 24 weeks)
PO	per oral
PR	per rectum
PV	per vagina
RDS	respiratory distress syndrome
ROA	right occipito anterior
ROP	right occipito posterior
SB	stillbirth
SCBU	special care baby unit
SGA	small for gestational age
SROM	spontaneous rupture of membranes
TDS	three times daily
TPR	temperature, pulse and respirations
TTN	transient tacypnoea of the newborn
U & E	urea and electrolytes
USS	ultrasound scan
UTI	urinary tract infection
VBAC	vaginal birth after caesarean
VE	vaginal examination
X match	cross match

Support groups

Citizen's advice bureau – 02078332181

Contact a Family – for parents with/expecting disabled children – 08088083555

Drinkline – 0800 9178282

FSA – Financial Services Authority – 08456061234

La Leche league – breastfeeding advice and support – 08451202918

Miscarriage Association – 01924200799

National Domestic Violence helpline – 080820000247

NCT – National Childbirth Trust – 03003300772

NHS Direct – 08454647

NHS Pregnancy Smoking Helpline – 08001699169

SANDS – Stillbirth and Neonatal Deaths – 02074365881

TAMBA – Twins and Multiple Births Association – 01483304442

Women at risk (FGM) – 02072019982

Working Families (Rights and benefits) – 08000130313

Shift roster

DAY	DATE	SHIFT
MONDAY		
TUESDAY		
WEDNESDAY		
THURSDAY		
FRIDAY		
SATURDAY		
SUNDAY		